THE PLANT BASED DIET COOKBOOK

50 Quick & Easy Affordable Recipes That Novice And Busy People Can Do, Cook Quick And Easy Wholesome Meals On A Totally Plant Based Ingredients

Elena Peterson

Table of Contents

INTRODUCTION..8

CHAPTER 1: BREAKFAST RECIPES 14

    1.   APPLE-WALNUT BREAKFAST BREAD..............................14
    2.   VEGAN SALMON BAGEL 16
    3.   MINT CHOCOLATE GREEN PROTEIN SMOOTHIE 17
    4.   DAIRY-FREE COCONUT YOGURT....................................18
    5.   VEGAN GREEN AVOCADO SMOOTHIE.............................19

CHAPTER 2: LUNCH RECIPES 20

    6.   SWEET POTATO AND QUINOA BOWL 20
    7.   CHICKPEA SALAD BITES..22
    8.   AVOCADO AND CHICKPEAS LETTUCE CUPS...................24
    9.   PESTO QUINOA WITH WHITE BEANS...............................26
    10.   GREEN BEAN CASSEROLE 28

CHAPTER 3: DINNER RECIPES 30

    11.   TOFU NUGGETS WITH BARBECUE GLAZE 30
    12.   PEPPERED PINTO BEANS 31
    13.   BLACK BEAN PIZZA 32
    14.   VEGETABLE AND CHICKPEA LOAF..................................33
    15.   THYME AND LEMON COUSCOUS 35
    16.   PESTO AND WHITE BEAN PASTA 36

CHAPTER 4: VEGETABLES RECIPES 38

    17.   MINTED PEAS...38

CHAPTER 5: PASTA & NOODLES 40

    18.   20 MINUTES VEGETARIAN PASTA 40

CHAPTER 6: DIP AND SPREAD RECIPES 42

    19.   CREAMY CUCUMBER YOGURT DIP.................................42

CHAPTER 7: SMOOTHIES AND BEVERAGES 44

    20.   MANGO AGUA FRESCA..44
    21.   LIGHT GINGER TEA 46

CHAPTER 8: SIDE DISHES **48**

   22.   Coconut Cauliflower Mix 48

CHAPTER 9: SOUPS AND STEWS **50**

   23.   Mushroom & Broccoli Soup 50
   24.   Creamy Cauliflower Pakora Soup 52
   25.   Garden Vegetable and Herb Soup 54
   26.   Avocado Green Soup 56

CHAPTER 10: BREAD RECIPES **58**

   27.   Strawberry Bread 58

CHAPTER 11: INSTANT POT **60**

   28.   Chocolate Walnut Oatmeal 60

CHAPTER 12: SAUCES, DRESSINGS, AND DIPS **62**

   29.   Homemade Chimichurri 62
   30.   Cilantro Coconut Pesto 64
   31.   Fresh Mango Salsa 65

CHAPTER 13: SALADS RECIPES **66**

   32.   Lentil, Lemon & Mushroom Salad 66

CHAPTER 14: SNACK AND SIDES **68**

   33.   Beetroot Hummus 68
   34.   Carrot and Sweet Potato Fritters 70
   35.   Black Bean Lime Dip 71

CHAPTER 15: ENTRÉES **72**

   36.   Veggie Hummus Wraps 72

CHAPTER 16: ASIAN RECIPES **74**

   37.   Keto-Vegan Chili 74

CHAPTER 17: NUTRIENT-PACKED PROTEIN SALAD RECIPES **76**

   38.   Rice & Tofu Salad 76

CHAPTER 18: FINGER FOOD **78**

   39.   Pumpernickel with Avocado 78

CHAPTER 19: FRUIT SALAD RECIPES................................**80**

40.   FALL FRUIT WITH CREAMY DRESSING 80

CHAPTER 20: GRAINS AND BEANS **82**

41.   NOODLE AND RICE PILAF..82
42.   EASY MILLET LOAF 83

CHAPTER 21: DRINKS..**84**

43.   TURMERIC LASSI 84
44.   BROWNIE BATTER ORANGE CHIA SHAKE 85
45.   SAFFRON PISTACHIO BEVERAGE 86

CHAPTER 22: DESSERTS **88**

46.   BANANA-ALMOND CAKE..88
47.   BANANA-COCONUT ICE CREAM 90
48.   COCONUT BUTTER CLOUDS COOKIES 91
49.   CHOCOMINT HAZELNUT BARS 93
50.   COCO-CINNAMON BALLS 95

CHAPTER 23: 2 WEEKS MEAL PLAN **98**

CONCLUSION **100**

INTRODUCTION

Aplant-based diet is a diet based primarily on whole plant foods. It is identical to the regular diet we're used to already, except that it leaves out foods that are not exclusively from plants. Hence, a plant-based diet does away with all types of animal-sourced foods, hydrogenated oils, refined sugars, and processed foods. A whole food plant-based diet comprises not just fruits and vegetables; it also consists of unprocessed or barely-processed oils with healthy monounsaturated fats (like extra-virgin olive oil), whole grains, legumes (essentially lentils and beans), seeds and nuts, as well as herbs and spices.

What makes a plant-based meal (or any meal) fun is the manner with which you make them; the seasoning process; and the combination process that contributes to a fantastic flavor and makes every meal unique and enjoyable. There are lots of delicious recipes (all plant-centered), which will prove helpful in when you intend making mouthwatering, healthy plant-based dishes for personal or household consumption. Provided you're eating these plant-based foods regularly, you'll have very problems with fat or diseases that result from bad dietary habits, and there would be no need for excessive calorie tracking.

Plant-based diet recipes are versatile; they range from colorful Salads to Lentil Stews, and Bean Burritos. The recipes also draw influences from around the globe, with Mexican, Chinese, European, Indian cuisines all part of the vast array of plant-based recipes available to choose from.

Why You Ought to Reduce Your Intake of Processed and Animal-Based Foods

You have likely heard over and over that processed food has adverse effects on your health. You might have also been told repeatedly to stay away from foods with lots of preservatives; nevertheless, nobody ever offered any genuine or concrete facts about why you ought to avoid these foods and why they are unsafe. Consequently, let us properly dissect it to help you properly comprehend why you ought to stay away from these healthy eating offenders.

They have massive habit-forming characteristics

Humans have a predisposition towards being addicted to some specific foods; however, the reality is that the fault is not wholly ours.

Every one of the unhealthy treats we relish now and then triggers the dopamine release in our brains. This creates a pleasurable effect in our brain, but the excitement is usually short-lived. The discharged dopamine additionally causes an attachment connection gradually, and this is the reason some people consistently go back to eat certain unhealthy foods even when they know it's unhealthy and unnecessary. You can get rid of this by taking out that inducement completely.

They are sugar-laden and plenteous in glucose-fructose syrup

Animal-based and processed foods are laden with refined sugars and glucose-fructose syrup which has almost no beneficial food nutrient. An ever-increasing number of studies are affirming what several people presumed from the start; that genetically modified foods bring about inflammatory bowel disease, which consequently makes it increasingly difficult for the body to assimilate essential nutrients. The disadvantages that result from your body being unable to assimilate essential nutrients from consumed foods rightly cannot be overemphasized. Processed and animal-based food products contain plenteous amounts of refined carbohydrates. Indeed, your body requires carbohydrates to give it the needed energy to run body capacities.

In any case, refining carbs dispenses with the fundamental supplements; in the way that refining entire grains disposes of the whole grain part. What remains, in the wake of refining, is what's considered as empty carbs or empty calories. These can negatively affect the metabolic system in your body by sharply increasing your blood sugar and insulin quantities.

They contain lots of synthetic ingredients

At the point when your body is taking in non-natural ingredients, it regards them as foreign substances. Your body treats them as a health threat. Your body isn't accustomed to identifying synthetic compounds like sucralose or these synthesized sugars. Hence, in defense of your health against this foreign "aggressor," your body does what it's capable of to safeguard your health. It sets off an immune reaction to tackle this "enemy" compound, which indirectly weakens your body's general disease alertness, making you susceptible to illnesses. The concentration and energy expended by your body in ensuring your immune system remain safe could instead be devoted somewhere else.

They contain constituent elements that set off an excitable reward sensation in your body

A part of processed and animal-based foods contain compounds like glucose-fructose syrup, monosodium glutamate, and specific food dyes that can trigger some addiction. They rouse your body to receive a benefit in return whenever you consume them. Monosodium glutamate, for example, is added to many store-bought baked foods. This additive slowly conditions your palates to relish the taste. It gets mental just by how your brain interrelates with your taste sensors. This reward-centric arrangement makes you crave it increasingly, which ends up exposing you to the danger of overconsuming calories.

For animal protein, usually, the expression "subpar" is used to allude to plant proteins since they generally have lower levels of essential amino acids as against animal-sourced protein. Nevertheless, what the vast majority don't know is that large amounts of essential amino acids can prove detrimental to your health. Let me break it down further for you.

Animal-Sourced Protein has no Fiber

In their pursuit to consume animal protein increasingly, the vast majority wind up dislodging the plant protein that was previously available in their body. Replacing the plant proteins with its animal variant is wrong because, in contrast to plant protein, animal proteins typically have fiber deficiency, phytonutrients, and antioxidant properties. Fiber insufficiency is a regular feature across various regions and societies on the planet. In America, for example, according to the National Academy of Medicine, the typical adult takes in roughly 15 grams of dietary fiber daily rather than the recommended daily quantity of 25 to 30 grams. A deficiency in dietary fiber often leads to a heightened risk of breast and colorectal cancers, in addition to constipation, inflammatory bowel disease, and cardiovascular disease.

Animal Protein Leads to a Jump in IGF-1 Levels

Insulin-like growth factor 1 (IGF-1) is a vital growth hormone identical in molecular geometry to insulin which contributes significantly to the growth of children and impacts adults in an anabolic manner. It fuels cell division and development, which may seemingly seem positive; however, it correspondingly triggers the development of cancer cells. Hence, an increased level of IGF-1 in the blood is connected to a heightened risk of cancer, malignant tumor, and spread.

Animal protein brings about an upsurge in Phosphorus levels in the body

Animal protein has significant levels of Phosphorus. Our bodies stabilize these plenteous amounts of Phosphorus by producing and discharging a hormone known as fibroblast growth factor 23 (FGF23). Studies have shown that this hormone is dangerous to our veins. FGF23 also causes asymmetrical expansion of heart muscles — a determinant for congestive heart failure and even mortality in some advanced cases.

Having discussed the many problems associated with animal protein, it becomes more apt to replace its "high quality" perception with the tag, "highly hazardous." In contrast to caffeine, which has a withdrawal effect if it's discontinued abruptly, you can stop taking processed and animal-based foods right away without any withdrawals. Possibly the only thing that you'll give up is the ease of some meals taking little-to-no time to prepare.

CHAPTER 1:

BREAKFAST RECIPES

1. Apple-Walnut Breakfast Bread

Preparation Time: 15 minutes

Cooking Time: 60 minutes

Servings: 8 servings

Ingredients:

- 1 1/2 cups apple sauce
- 1/3 cup plant milk
- 2 cups all-purpose flour
- Salt to taste
- 1 teaspoon ground cinnamon
- 1 tablespoon flax seeds mixed with 2 tablespoons warm water
- 3/4 cup brown sugar
- 1 teaspoon baking powder
- 1/2 cup chopped walnuts

Directions:

1. Preheat to 375 degree Fahrenheit.
2. Combine the apple sauce, sugar, milk, and flax mixture in a jar and mix.

3. Combine the flour, baking powder, salt, and cinnamon in a separate bowl.

4. Simply add dry **Ingredients:** into the wet **Ingredients:** and combine to make slices.

5. Bake for 25 minutes until it becomes light brown.

Nutrition: Calories: 309 Fat: 9.1g Carbohydrates: 16.5g Protein: 6.9g

2. Vegan Salmon Bagel

Preparation Time: 10 minutes

Cooking Time: 30 minutes

Servings: 2 servings

Ingredients:

- 4 cups of water
- 11/2 red onion
- Vegan cream cheese
- Salt, pepper
- 4 bagels
- 11/2 cup of apple cider vinegar
- 7 carrots

Directions:

1. Preheat to 200 degree Celsius.
2. Slice the carrots.
3. In a mixer to mix, combine sugar, vinegar, and ground pepper.
4. Put the carrot strips in a stir fry bowl, apply the marinade and stir.
5. Cover the carrots with foil and bake for twenty minutes, then switch heat down to 210°F and cook for 40 minutes more.

Nutrition: Calories: 232 Fat: 9.1g Carbohydrates: 71.5g Protein: 7.9g

3. **Mint Chocolate Green Protein Smoothie**

Preparation Time: 5 minutes

Cooking Time: 10 minutes

Servings: 1 servings

Ingredients:

- 1 scoop chocolate powder
- 1 tablespoon flaxseed
- 1 banana
- 1 mint leaf
- 3/4 cup almond milk
- 3 tablespoons dark chocolate (chopped)

Directions:

1. Blend all the **Ingredients:** except the dark chocolate.
2. Garnish dark chocolate when ready.

Nutrition: Calories: 300 Fat: 19.1g Carbohydrates: 21.5g Protein: 27.9g

4. Dairy-Free Coconut Yogurt

Preparation Time: 5 minutes

Cooking Time: 10 minutes

Servings: 2 servings

Ingredients:

- 1 can coconut milk

- 4 vegan probiotic capsules

Directions:

1. Shake coconut milk with a whole tube.

2. Remove the plastic of capsules and mix in.

3. Cut a 12-inch cheesecloth until stirred.

4. Freeze or eat immediately.

Nutrition: Calories: 219 Fat: 10.1g Carbohydrates: 1.5g Protein: 7.9g

5.   <u>Vegan Green Avocado Smoothie</u>

Preparation Time: 5 minutes

Cooking Time: 10 minutes

Servings: 2 servings

Ingredients:

- 1 banana

- 1 cup water

- 1/2 avocado

- 1/2 lemon juice

- 1/2 cup coconut yoghurt

Directions:

1. Blend all **Ingredients:** until smooth.

Nutrition: Calories: 299 Fat: 1.1g Carbohydrates: 1.5g Protein: 7.9g

CHAPTER 2:

LUNCH RECIPES

6.   Sweet Potato and Quinoa Bowl

Preparation Time: 5 minutes

Cooking Time: 20 minutes

Servings: 4

Ingredients:

- 2 cups quinoa
- 1 cup diced red onion
- 2 cups diced sweet potato
- 1 1/2 cup raisins
- 1 cup sunflower seeds, shelled, unsalted
- 2 cups vegetable broth

Directions:

1. Take a medium pot, place it over high heat, add quinoa, and sweet potatoes, pour in vegetable broth, stir until mixed and bring it to a boil.

2. Then switch heat to medium-low level, cover pot with the lid, and cook for 20 minutes until the quinoa has cooked.

3. When done, remove the pot from heat and fluff quinoa by using a fork.

4. Add onion, raisins, and sunflower seeds, stir until mixed and transfer into a large bowl.

5. Let it chill in the refrigerator for 30 minutes and then serve.

Nutrition: 204 Cal 7 g Fat 3 g Saturated Fat 31 g Carbohydrates 3 g Fiber 11 g Sugars 3 g Protein;

7.   Chickpea Salad Bites

Preparation Time: 15 minutes

Cooking Time: 0 minutes

Servings: 4

Ingredients:

For the Bread:

- 2 tablespoons chopped parsley
- 1 small green chili pepper
- 1/3 cup of raisins
- 1 teaspoon garlic powder
- ½ teaspoon salt
- 1/3 teaspoon ground black pepper
- ½ teaspoon smoked paprika
- ½ tablespoon maple syrup
- ½ teaspoon cayenne pepper
- 2 tablespoons balsamic vinegar
- 1 1/2 cups crumbled rye bread, whole-grain

For the Salad:

- 2 scallions, chopped
- 1/3 cup chopped pickles
- 2 tablespoons chopped chives and more for topping
- ½ teaspoon minced garlic
- 1 ½ cup cooked chickpeas
- 1 lemon, juiced

- ½ teaspoon salt
- ¼ teaspoon ground black pepper
- 1 tablespoons poppy seeds
- 1 teaspoon mustard paste
- 1/3 cup coconut yogurt

Directions:

1. Prepare the bread, and for this, place all of its ingredients in a food processor and then pulse for 1 minute until just combined; don't overmix.
2. Then make bites of the bread mixture and for this, take a 2.3-inch round cookie cutter, add 2 tablespoons of the bread mixture, press it into the cutter, and gently lift it out, repeat with the remaining batter to make seven more bites.
3. Prepare the salad and for this, take a large bowl, add chickpeas in it, then add chives, scallion, pickles, and garlic and then mash chickpeas by using a fork until broken.
4. Add remaining ingredients for the salad and stir until well mixed.
5. Assemble the bites and for this, top each prepared bread bite generously with prepared salad, sprinkle with chives and poppy seeds, and then serve.

Nutrition: 210 Cal 4 g Fat 1 g Saturated Fat 36 g Carbohydrates 6 g Fiber 4 g Sugars 7 g Protein;

8. Avocado and Chickpeas Lettuce Cups

Preparation Time: 10 minutes

Cooking Time: 0 minutes

Servings: 4

Ingredients:

- 2 small avocados, peeled, pitted, diced
- 8 ounces hearts of palm
- ¾ cup cooked chickpeas
- 1/2 cup cucumber, diced
- 1 tablespoon minced shallots
- 2 cups mixed greens
- 1 tablespoon Dijon mustard
- 1 lime, zested, juiced
- 2 tablespoons chopped cilantro and more for topping
- 2/3 teaspoon salt
- 1/3 teaspoon ground black pepper
- 1 tablespoon apple cider vinegar
- 2 ½ tablespoons olive oil

Directions:

1. Take a medium bowl, add shallots and cilantro in it, stir in salt, black pepper, mustard, vinegar, lime juice, and zest until just mixed and then slowly mix in olive oil until combined.

2. Add cucumber, hearts of palm and chickpeas, stir until mixed, fold in avocado and then top with some more cilantro.

3. Distribute mixed greens among four plates, top with chickpea mixture and then serve.

Nutrition: 280 Cal 12.6 g Fat 1.5 g Saturated Fat 32.8 g Carbohydrates 9.3 g Fiber 1.2 g Sugars 7.6 g Protein;

9. Pesto Quinoa with White Beans

Preparation Time: 5 minutes

Cooking Time: 15 minutes

Servings: 4

Ingredients:

- 12 ounces cooked white bean
- 3 ½ cups quinoa, cooked
- 1 medium zucchini, sliced
- ¾ cup sun-dried tomato
- ¼ cup pine nuts
- 1 tablespoon olive oil

For the Pesto:

- 1/3 cup walnuts
- 2 cups arugula
- 1 teaspoon minced garlic
- 2 cups basil
- ¾ teaspoon salt
- ¼ teaspoon ground black pepper
- 1 tablespoon lemon juice
- 1/3 cup olive oil
- 2 tablespoons water

Directions:

1. Prepare the pesto, and for this, place all of its ingredients in a food processor and pulse for 2 minutes

until smooth, scraping the sides of the container frequently and set aside until required.

2. Take a large skillet pan, place it over medium heat, add oil and when hot, add zucchini and cook for 4 minutes until tender-crisp.

3. Season zucchini with salt and black pepper, cook for 2 minutes until lightly brown, then add tomatoes and white beans and continue cooking for 4 minutes until white beans begin to crisp.

4. Stir in pine nuts, cook for 2 minutes until toasted, then remove the pan from heat and transfer zucchini mixture into a medium bowl.

5. Add quinoa and pesto, stir until well combined, then distribute among four bowls and then serve.

Nutrition: 352 Cal 27.3 g Fat 5 g Saturated Fat 33.7 g Carbohydrates 5.7 g Fiber 4.5 g Sugars 9.7 g Protein;

10.   Green Bean Casserole

Preparation Time: 5 minutes

Cooking Time: 40 minutes

Servings: 4

Ingredients:

- 6 ounces fried onions
- 1 ½ cups cremini mushrooms, diced
- 16 ounces frozen green beans
- ½ cup diced white onion
- 1 tablespoon minced garlic
- 3 ½ tablespoons all-purpose flour
- 1/3 teaspoon ground black pepper
- ½ teaspoon dried oregano
- 3 ½ tablespoons olive oil
- 2 cups vegetable broth, hot

Directions:

1. Switch on the oven, then set it to 400 degrees F and let it preheat.

2. Take a medium saucepan, place it over medium heat, add oil and when hot, add onion and mushrooms, stir in garlic and cook for 4 minutes until tender.

3. Stir in flour until the thick paste comes together and then cook for 2 minutes until golden.

4. Stir in vegetable broth, bring it to a simmer, then stir in black pepper and oregano, whisk well and cook for 15 minutes until gravy thickened to the desired level.

5. Add green beans, stir until mixed, remove the pan from heat, top beans with fried onions and bake for 15 minutes.

6. Serve straight away.

Nutrition: 191 Cal 10 g Fat 2 g Saturated Fat 22 g Carbohydrates 3.3 g Fiber 2.5 g Sugars 4.1 g Protein;

CHAPTER 3:

DINNER RECIPES

11.   Tofu Nuggets with Barbecue Glaze

Preparation Time: 10 minutes

Cooking Time: 25 minutes

Servings: 9

Ingredients:

- 32 ounces tofu
- 1 cup quick vegan barbecue sauce

Directions:

1. Set the oven to 425F.
2. Next, slice the tofu and blot the tofu with clean towels. Next, slice and dice the tofu and completely eliminate the water from the tofu material.
3. Stir the tofu with the vegan barbecue sauce, and place the tofu on a baking sheet.
4. Bake the tofu for fifteen minutes. Afterward, stir the tofu and bake the tofu for an additional ten minutes.
5. Enjoy!

Nutrition: Calories: 311 kcal Protein: 19.94 g Fat: 21.02 g Carbohydrates: 15.55 g

12.   Peppered Pinto Beans

Preparation Time: 10 minutes

Cooking Time: 15 minutes

Servings: 6

Ingredients:

- 1 tsp. Chili powder
- 1 tsp. ground cumin
- .5 cup Vegetable
- 2 cans Pinto beans
- 1 Minced jalapeno
- 1 Diced red bell pepper
- 1 tsp. Olive oil

Directions:

1. Take out a pot and heat the oil. Cook the jalapeno and pepper for a bit before adding in the pepper, salt, cumin, broth, and beans.

2. Place to a boil and then reduce the heat to cook for a bit. After 10 minutes, let it cool and serve.

Nutrition: Calories: 183 Carbs: 32g Fat: 2g Protein: 11g

13. **Black Bean Pizza**

Preparation Time: 30 minutes

Cooking Time: 20 minutes

Servings: 2

Ingredients:

- 1 Sliced avocado
- 1 Sliced red onion
- 1 Grated carrot
- 1 Sliced tomato
- .5 cup Spicy black bean dip
- 2 Pizza crusts

Directions:

1. Turn on the oven and let heat to 400 degrees. Layout two crusts on a baking sheet and add the dip onto each one.

2. Top with the tomato slices and sprinkle the carrots and the onion on a well.

3. Add to the oven and let it bake for about 20 minutes or so until done. Top with the avocado before serving.

Nutrition: Calories: 379 Carbs: 59g Fat: 13g Protein: 13g

14.   Vegetable and Chickpea Loaf

Preparation Time: 10 minutes

Cooking Time: 15 minutes

Servings: 4

Ingredients:

- 1 tsp. Salt
- .5 tsp. Dried sage
- 1 tsp. Dried savory
- 1 tbsp. Soy sauce
- .25 cup Parsley
- .5 cup Breadcrumbs
- .75 cup Oats
- .75 cup Chickpea flour
- 1.5 cup cooked chickpeas
- 2 Minced garlic cloves
- 1 Chopped yellow onion
- 1 Shredded carrot
- 1 Shredded white potato

Directions:

1. Set the oven to 350F. Take out a loaf pan and then grease it up.

2. Squeeze out the liquid from the potato and add to the food processor with the garlic, onion, and carrot.

3. Add the chickpeas and pulse to blend well. Add in the rest of the ingredients here, and when it is done, use your hands to form this into a loaf and add to the pan.

4. Place into the oven to bake for a bit until it is nice and firm. Let it cool down and then slice.

Nutrition: Calories: 351 kcal Protein: 16.86 g Fat: 6.51 g Carbohydrates: 64 g

15.   Thyme and Lemon Couscous

Preparation Time: 5 minutes

Cooking Time: 10 minutes

Servings: 6

Ingredients:

- .25 cup Chopped parsley
- 1.5 cup Couscous
- 2 tbsp. Chopped thyme
- Juice and zest of a lemon
- 2.75 cup Vegetable stock

Directions:

1. Take out a pot and add in the thyme, lemon juice, and vegetable stock. Stir in the couscous after it has gotten to a boil and then take off the heat.
2. Allow sitting covered until it can take in all of the liquid. Then fluff up with a form.
3. Stir in the parsley and lemon zest, then serve warm.

Nutrition: Calories: 922 kcal Protein: 2.7 g Fat: 101.04 g Carbohydrates: 10.02 g

16.   Pesto and White Bean Pasta

Preparation Time: 10 minutes

Cooking Time: 10 minutes

Servings: 4

Ingredients:

- .5 cup Chopped black olives
- .25 Diced red onion
- 1 cup Chopped tomato
- .5 cup Spinach pesto
- 1.5 cup Cannellini beans
- 8 oz. Rotini pasta, cooked

Directions:

1. Bring out a bowl and toss together the pesto, beans, and pasta.
2. Add in the olives, red onion, and tomato and toss around a bit more before serving.

Nutrition: Calories 544 Carbs 83g Fat 17g Protein 23g

CHAPTER 4:

VEGETABLES RECIPES

17.   Minted Peas

Preparation Time: 5 minutes

Cooking Time: 5 minutes

Servings: 4

Ingredients:

- 1 tablespoon olive oil
- 4 cups peas, fresh or frozen (not canned)
- ½ teaspoon sea salt
- freshly ground black pepper
- 3 tablespoons chopped fresh mint

Directions:

1. In a large sauté pan, heat the olive oil over medium-high heat until hot. Add the peas and cook, about 5 minutes.
2. Remove the pan from heat. Stir in the salt, season with pepper, and stir in the mint.
3. Serve hot.

Nutrition: Calories: 77 Fat: 3g Protein: 4g Carbohydrates: 12g Fiber: 5g Sugar: 3g Sodium: 320mg

CHAPTER 5:

PASTA & NOODLES

18.   20 Minutes Vegetarian Pasta

Preparation Time: 5 minutes

Cooking Time: 16 minutes

Servings: 4

Ingredients:

- 3 shallots, chopped
- ¼ teaspoon red pepper flakes
- ¼ cup vegan parmesan cheese
- 2 tablespoons olive oil
- 2 garlic cloves, minced
- 8-ounces spinach leaves
- 8-ounces linguine pasta
- 1 pinch salt
- 1 pinch black pepper

Directions:

1. Boil salted water in a large pot and add pasta.
2. Cook for about 6 minutes and drain the pasta in a colander.
3. Heat olive oil over medium heat in a large skillet and add the shallots.

4. Cook for about 5 minutes until soft and caramelized and stir in the spinach, garlic, red pepper flakes, salt and black pepper.

5. Cook for about 5 minutes and add pasta and 2 ladles of pasta water.

6. Stir in the parmesan cheese and dish out in a bowl to serve.

Nutrition: Calories: 284 Total Fat: 18g Protein: 29g Total Carbs: 1.5g Fiber: 0g Net Carbs: 1.5g

CHAPTER 6:

DIP AND SPREAD RECIPES

19.   Creamy Cucumber Yogurt Dip

Preparation Time: 15 minutes

Cooking Time: 15 minutes

Servings: 4

Ingredients:

- 1 cup (8 oz.) reduced-fat plain yogurt
- 4 oz. reduced-fat cream cheese
- 1/2 cup chopped seeded peeled cucumber
- 1-1/2 teaspoon. finely chopped onion
- 1-1/2 teaspoon. snipped fresh dill or 1/2 teaspoon dill weed
- 1 teaspoon lemon juice
- 1 teaspoon grated lemon peel
- 1 garlic clove, minced
- 1/4 teaspoon salt
- 1/4 teaspoon pepper
- Assorted fresh vegetables

Directions:

1. Mix the cream cheese and yogurt in a small bowl. Stir in pepper, salt, garlic, peel, lemon juice, dill, onion, and

cucumber. Put on the cover and let it chill in the fridge. Serve it with the veggies.

Nutrition: calories 55 fat 4 carbs 12 protein 6

CHAPTER 7:

SMOOTHIES AND BEVERAGES

20.   Mango Agua Fresca

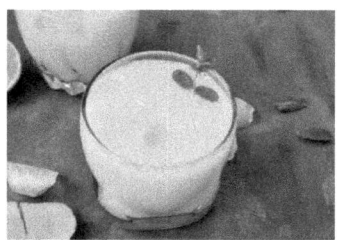

Preparation Time: 5 minutes

Cooking Time: 0 minutes

Servings: 2

Ingredients:

- 2 fresh mangoes, diced
- 1½ cups water
- 1 teaspoon fresh lime juice
- Maple syrup, to taste
- 2 cups ice
- 2 slices fresh lime, for garnish
- 2 fresh mint sprigs, for garnish

Directions:

1. Put the mangoes, lime juice, maple syrup, and water in a blender. Process until creamy and smooth.

2. Divide the beverage into two glasses, then garnish each glass with ice, lime slice, and mint sprig before serving.

Nutrition: calories: 230 fat: 1.3g carbs: 57.7g fiber: 5.4g protein: 2.8g

21.   Light Ginger Tea

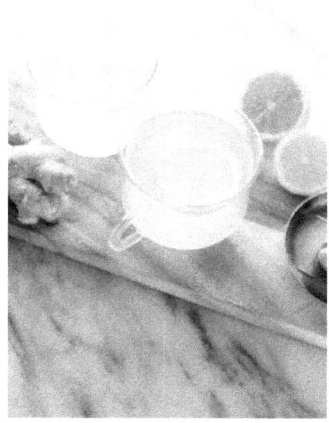

Preparation Time: 5 minutes

Cooking Time: 10 to 15 minutes

Servings: 2

Ingredients:

- 1 small ginger knob, sliced into four 1-inch chunks
- 4 cups water
- Juice of 1 large lemon
- Maple syrup, to taste

Directions:

1. Add the ginger knob and water in a saucepan, then simmer over medium heat for 10 to 15 minutes.
2. Turn off the heat, then mix in the lemon juice. Strain the liquid to remove the ginger, then fold in the maple syrup and serve.

Nutrition: calories: 32 fat: 0.1g carbs: 8.6g fiber: 0.1g protein: 0.1g

CHAPTER 8:

SIDE DISHES

22.   Coconut Cauliflower Mix

Time: 10 minutes **Cooking Time:** 10 minutes **Servings:** 6

Ingredients:

- 1 pound cauliflower florets
- 1 cup of water
- 1/4 cup of coconut milk
- 1 tablespoon coconut yogurt
- 1 teaspoon salt
- 1 teaspoon hot paprika
- 1 teaspoon Italian seasoning
- 1 tablespoon chives, chopped

Directions:

1. Place cauliflower and water in the instant pot. Add salt and close the lid.
2. Cook the vegetables on Manual mode for 10 minutes.
3. Then use quick pressure release.
4. Open the lid, drain water and mash the cauliflower.
5. Add the rest of the Ingredients, stir well and serve.

Nutrition: Calories: 211, Fat: 4.6, Fiber: 5.3, Carbs: 24.2, Protein: 3.9

CHAPTER 9:

SOUPS AND STEWS

23. <u>Mushroom & Broccoli Soup</u>

Preparation Time: 20 minutes

Cooking Time: 45 minutes

Servings: 8

Ingredients:

- 1 bundle broccoli (around 1-1/2 pounds)
- 1 tablespoon canola oil
- 1/2 pound cut crisp mushrooms
- 1 tablespoon diminished sodium soy sauce
- 2 medium carrots, finely slashed
- 2 celery ribs, finely slashed
- 1/4 cup finely slashed onion
- 1 garlic clove, minced
- 1 container (32 ounces) vegetable juices
- 2 cups of water
- 2 tablespoons lemon juice

Directions:

1. Cut broccoli florets into reduced down pieces. Strip and hack stalks.

2. In an enormous pot, heat oil over medium-high warmth; saute mushrooms until delicate, 4-6 minutes. Mix in soy sauce; expel from skillet.

3. In the same container, join broccoli stalks, carrots, celery, onion, garlic, soup, and water; heat to the point of boiling. Diminish heat; stew, revealed, until vegetables are relaxed, 25-30 minutes.

4. Puree soup utilizing a drenching blender. Or then again, cool marginally and puree the soup in a blender; come back to the dish.

5. Mix in florets and mushrooms; heat to the point of boiling. Lessen warmth to medium; cook until broccoli is delicate, 8-10 minutes, blending infrequently. Mix in lemon juice.

Nutrition: kcal: 830 Carbohydrates: 8 g Protein: 45 g Fat: 64 g

24.   <u>Creamy Cauliflower Pakora Soup</u>

Preparation Time: 20 minutes

Cooking Time: 20 minutes

Servings: 8

Ingredients:

- 1 huge head cauliflower, cut into little florets
- 5 medium potatoes, stripped and diced
- 1 huge onion, diced
- 4 medium carrots, stripped and diced
- 2 celery ribs, diced
- 1 container (32 ounces) vegetable stock
- 1 teaspoon garam masala
- 1 teaspoon garlic powder
- 1 teaspoon ground coriander
- 1 teaspoon ground turmeric
- 1 teaspoon ground cumin
- 1 teaspoon pepper
- 1 teaspoon salt
- 1/2 teaspoon squashed red pepper chips
- Water or extra vegetable stock
- New cilantro leaves
- Lime wedges, discretionary

Directions:

1. In a Dutch stove over medium-high warmth, heat initial 14 fixings to the point of boiling. Cook and mix until vegetables

are delicate, around 20 minutes. Expel from heat; cool marginally. Procedure in groups in a blender or nourishment processor until smooth. Modify consistency as wanted with water (or extra stock). Sprinkle with new cilantro. Serve hot, with lime wedges whenever wanted.

2. Stop alternative: Before including cilantro, solidify cooled soup in cooler compartments. To utilize, in part defrost in cooler medium-term.

3. Warmth through in a pan, blending every so often and including a little water if fundamental. Sprinkle with cilantro. Whenever wanted, present with lime wedges.

Nutrition: kcal: 248 Carbohydrates: 7 g Protein: 1 g Fat: 19 g

25.   Garden Vegetable and Herb Soup

Preparation Time: 20 minutes

Cooking Time: 30 minutes

Servings: 8

Ingredients:

- 2 tablespoons olive oil
- 2 medium onions, hacked
- 2 huge carrots, cut
- 1 pound red potatoes (around 3 medium), cubed
- 2 cups of water
- 1 can (14-1/2 ounces) diced tomatoes in sauce
- 1-1/2 cups vegetable soup
- 1-1/2 teaspoons garlic powder
- 1 teaspoon dried basil
- 1/2 teaspoon salt
- 1/2 teaspoon paprika
- 1/4 teaspoon dill weed
- 1/4 teaspoon pepper
- 1 medium yellow summer squash, split and cut
- 1 medium zucchini, split and cut

Directions:

1. In a huge pan, heat oil over medium warmth. Include onions and carrots; cook and mix until onions are delicate, 4-6 minutes. Include potatoes and cook 2 minutes. Mix in water, tomatoes, juices, and seasonings.

2. Heat to the point of boiling. Diminish heat; stew, revealed, until potatoes and carrots are delicate, 9 minutes.

3. Include yellow squash and zucchini; cook until vegetables are delicate, 9 minutes longer. Serve or, whenever wanted, puree blend in clusters, including extra stock until desired consistency is accomplished.

Nutrition: kcal: 252 Carbohydrates: 12 g Protein: 1 g Fat: 11 g

26. Avocado Green Soup

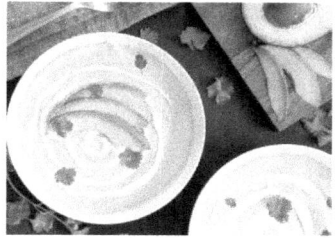

Preparation Time: 5 Minutes

Cooking Time: 5 Minutes

Servings: 4

Ingredients:

- 2 tbsp olive oil
- 1 ½ cup fresh kale, chopped coarsely
- 1 ½ cup fresh spinach, chopped coarsely
- 3 large avocados, halved, pitted and pulp extracted
- 2 cups of soy milk
- 2 cups no-sodium vegetable broth
- 3 tbsp chopped fresh mint leaves
- ¼ tsp salt
- ¼ tsp black pepper
- 2 limes, juiced

Directions:

1. Heat the olive oil in a medium saucepan over medium heat and mix in the kale and spinach. Cook until wilted, 3 minutes and turn off the heat.

2. Add the remaining ingredients and using an immersion blender, puree the soup until smooth.

3. Dish the soup and serve immediately.

Nutrition: Calories 400 Fat 10 g Protein 20 g Carbohydrates 30 g

CHAPTER 10:

BREAD RECIPES

27.   Strawberry Bread

Preparation Time: 15 Minutes

Cooking Time: 60 Minutes

Servings: 10

Ingredients:

- All-purpose flour – 2 cups
- Vanilla – 1 teaspoon.
- Vegetable oil – 1/2 cup
- Baking soda – 1 teaspoon.
- Cinnamon – 1/2 teaspoon.
- Brown sugar – 1/2 cup
- White sugar – 1/2 cup
- Fresh strawberries – 2 1/4 cups, chopped
- Salt – 1/2 teaspoon.

Directions:

1. Preheat the oven to 350 F. Grease 9.5-inch loaf pan and set aside.
2. In a mixing bowl, mix together flour, baking soda, cinnamon, brown sugar, white sugar, and salt.
3. In a separate bowl, vanilla, and oil. Stir in strawberries.

4. Add flour mixture to the strawberries mixture and stir until well combined.

5. Pour batter into the prepared loaf pan and bake in preheated oven for 50-60 minutes.

6. Allow to cool for 10-15 minutes. Slice and serve.

Nutrition: Calories 364, Carbs 40.1g, Fat 21.g, Protein 4.2g

CHAPTER 11:

INSTANT POT

28.   Chocolate Walnut Oatmeal

Time: 15 minutes **Cooking Time:** 5 minutes **Servings:** 2

Ingredients:

- 1/2 cup steel-cut oats
- 2 tablespoons cocoa powder
- 1 teaspoon brown sugar
- 1 tablespoon agave nectar
- 1 teaspoon vanilla extract
- 1/2 cup unsweetened almond milk
- 1 1/2 cups water
- Semi-sweet chocolate chips, for topping
- Walnuts for topping

Directions:

1. Spray the instant pot with nonstick spray. Combine the oats, cocoa powder, water, vanilla, brown sugar, and agave nectar.

2. Cook on high 3 minutes, then let the pressure release naturally. Stir in the almond milk.

3. Top with chocolate chips and walnuts.

Nutrition: Calories: 275 Fat: 16.5 Fiber: 4.3 Carbs: 17.2 Protein: 17.4

CHAPTER 12:

SAUCES, DRESSINGS, AND DIPS

29.   <u>Homemade Chimichurri</u>

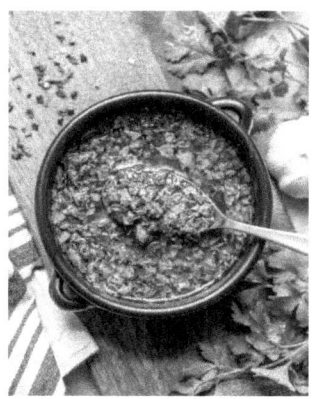

Preparation Time: 5 minutes **Cooking Time:** 0 minutes

Servings: 1

Ingredients:

- 1 cup finely chopped flat-leaf parsley leaves
- Zest and juice of 2 lemons
- ¼ cup low-sodium vegetable broth
- 4 garlic cloves
- 1 teaspoon dried oregano

Directions:

1. Place all the ingredients into a food processor, and pulse until it reaches the consistency you like.

2. Refrigerate the chimichurri in an airtight container for up to 5 days. It's best served within 1 day.

Nutrition: calories: 19 fat: 0.2g carbs: 3.7g protein: 0.7g fiber: 0.7g

30.   Cilantro Coconut Pesto

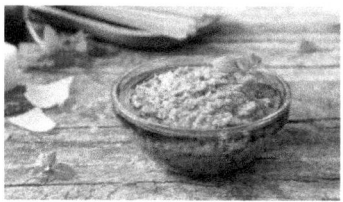

Preparation Time: 5 minutes

Cooking Time: 0 minutes

Servings: 2

Ingredients:

- 1 (13.5-ounce / 383-g) can unsweetened coconut milk
- 2 jalapeños, seeds and ribs removed
- 1 bunch cilantro, leaves only
- 1 tablespoon white miso
- 1-inch (2.5 cm) piece ginger, peeled and minced
- Water, as needed

Directions:

1. Pulse all the ingredients in a blender until creamy and smooth.
2. Thin with a little extra water as needed to reach your preferred consistency.
3. Store in an airtight container in the fridge for up t0 2 days or in the freezer for up to 6 months.

Nutrition: calories: 141 fat: 13.7g carbs: 2.8g protein: 1.6g fiber: 0.3g

31.   Fresh Mango Salsa

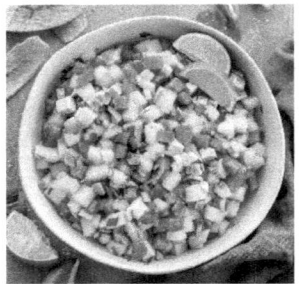

Preparation Time: 10 minutes

Cooking Time: 0 minutes

Servings: 6

Ingredients:

- 2 small mangoes, diced
- 1 red bell pepper, finely diced
- ½ red onion, finely diced
- Juice of ½ lime, or more to taste
- 2 tablespoon low-sodium vegetable broth
- Handful cilantro, chopped
- Freshly ground black pepper, to taste
- Salt, to taste (optional)

Directions:

1. Stir together all the ingredients in a large bowl until well incorporated.
2. Taste and add more lime juice or salt, if needed.
3. Store in an airtight container in the fridge for up to 5 days.

Nutrition: calories: 86 fat: 1.9g carbs: 13.3g protein: 1.2g fiber: 0.9g

CHAPTER 13:

SALADS RECIPES

32.   <u>Lentil, Lemon & Mushroom Salad</u>

Preparation Time: 10 minutes **Cooking Time:** 0 minutes

Servings: 2

Ingredients:

- ½ cup dry lentils of choice
- 2 cups vegetable broth
- 3 cups mushrooms, thickly sliced
- 1 cup sweet or purple onion, chopped
- 4 tsp. extra virgin olive oil
- 2 tbsp. garlic powder
- ¼ tsp. chili flakes
- 1 tbsp. lemon juice
- 2 tbsp. cilantro, chopped
- ½ cup arugula
- ¼ tsp Salt
- ¼ tsp pepper

Directions:

1. Sprout the lentils according the method. (Don't cook them).

2. Place the vegetable stock in a deep saucepan and bring it to a boil.

3. Add the lentils to the boiling broth, cover the pan, and cook for about 5 minutes over low heat until the lentils are a bit tender.

4. Remove the pan from heat and drain the excess water.

5. Put a frying pan over high heat and add 2 tablespoons of olive oil.

6. Add the onions, garlic, and chili flakes, and cook until the onions are almost translucent, around 5 to 10 minutes while stirring.

7. Add the mushrooms to the frying pan and mix in thoroughly. Continue cooking until the onions are completely translucent and the mushrooms have softened; remove the pan from the heat.

8. Mix the lentils, onions, mushrooms, and garlic in a large bowl.

9. Add the lemon juice and the remaining olive oil. Toss or stir to combine everything thoroughly.

10. Serve the mushroom/onion mixture over some arugala in bowl, adding salt and pepper to taste, or, store and enjoy later!

Nutrition: Calories 365 Total Fat 11.7g Saturated Fat 1.9g Cholesterol 0mg Sodium 1071mg Total Carbohydrate 45.2g Dietary Fiber 18g Total Sugars 8.2g Protein 22.8g Vitamin D 378mcg Calcium 67mg Iron 8mg Potassium 1212mg

CHAPTER 14:

SNACK AND SIDES

33.   Beetroot Hummus

Total time: 70 minutes

Ingredients

- 15 ounces cooked chickpeas
- 3 small beets
- 1 teaspoon minced garlic
- 1/2 teaspoon smoked paprika
- 1 teaspoon of sea salt
- 1/4 teaspoon red chili flakes
- 2 tablespoons olive oil
- 1 lemon, juiced
- 2 tablespoon tahini
- 1 tablespoon chopped almonds
- 1 tablespoon chopped cilantro

Directions:

1. Drizzle oil over beets, season with salt, then wrap beets in a foil and bake for 60 minutes at 425 degrees F until tender.

2. When done, let beet cool for 10 minutes, then peel and dice them and place them in a food processor.

3. Add remaining ingredients and pulse for 2 minutes until smooth, tip the hummus in a bowl, drizzle with some more oil, and then serve straight away.

34.   <u>Carrot and Sweet Potato Fritters</u>

Total time: 18 minutes

Ingredients

- 1/3 cup quinoa flour
- 1½ cups shredded sweet potato
- 1 cup grated carrot
- 1/3 teaspoon ground black pepper
- 2/3 teaspoon salt
- 2 teaspoons curry powder
- 2 flax eggs
- 2 tablespoons coconut oil

Directions:

1. Place all the ingredients in a bowl, except for oil, stir well until combined and then shape the mixture into ten small patties

2. Take a large pan, place it over medium-high heat, add oil and when it melts, add patties in it and cook for 3 minutes per side until browned.

3. Serve straight away

35.   <u>Black Bean Lime Dip</u>

Total time: 11 minutes

Ingredients

- 15.5 ounces cooked black beans
- 1 teaspoon minced garlic
- ½ of a lime, juiced
- 1 inch of ginger, grated
- 1/3 teaspoon salt
- 1/3 teaspoon ground black pepper
- 1 tablespoon olive oil

Directions:

1. Take a frying pan, add oil and when hot, add garlic and ginger and cook for 1 minute until fragrant.
2. Then add beans, splash with some water and fry for 3 minutes until hot.
3. Season beans with salt and black pepper, drizzle with lime juice, then remove the pan from heat and mash the beans until smooth pasta comes together.
4. Serve the dip with whole-grain breadsticks or vegetables.

CHAPTER 15:

ENTRÉES

36.   <u>Veggie Hummus Wraps</u>

Time: 10 minutes   **Cooking Time:** 6 minutes   **Servings:** 2

Ingredients:

- Zucchini, peeled, sliced lengthwise into .25-inch-thick strips – 1
- Sea salt - .5 teaspoon
- Tomato, sliced – 1
- Kale, chopped – 1 cup
- Red onion, sliced - .125 cup
- Avocado, sliced – 1
- Olive oil – 1 tablespoon
- Black pepper, ground - .25 teaspoon
- Apple cider vinegar – 2 teaspoons
- Water – 1 tablespoon
- Hummus - .25 cup
- Whole-wheat tortillas, large – 2

Directions: Heat a large non-stick skillet or grill pan on the stove over medium heat. Meanwhile, coat the sliced zucchini with the olive oil, ground black pepper, and sea salt.

1. Place the seasoned zucchini on the preheated pan and let it cook on the first side for three minutes, flip it over, and cook for an additional two minutes. Remove the zucchini from the heat of the stove and set it aside.

2. Set the whole-wheat tortillas in the hot pan and allow them to toast for a minute. You want the tortillas to be lightly toasted, warm, and easy to wrap without tearing.

3. Combine the apple cider vinegar and water, then toss the avocado in the mixture. This will help prevent the avocado from browning. Drain off any excess liquid.

4. Divide the ingredients in half, so that you can fill both tortillas with an even amount of ingredients. To prepare spread the hummus down the center of the warm tortilla, top with the zucchini, tomato, red onion, kale, and avocado.

5. Wrap in the ends of the tortillas and then tightly wrap the sides around the filling. By folding it this way, you will prevent the filling from falling out. Serve immediately or store in the fridge until lunchtime.

Nutrition: Number of Calories in Individual **Servings:** 438 Protein Grams: 9 Fat Grams: 28 Total Carbohydrates Grams: 40 Net Carbohydrates Grams: 36

CHAPTER 16:

ASIAN RECIPES

37.   <u>Keto-Vegan Chili</u>

Preparation Time: 10-15 minutes

Cooking Time: 41 minutes

Servings: 6

Ingredients:

- 1 tablespoon cocoa powder, unsweetened 1 c. raw walnuts

- 16 oz. tofu, extra firm

- 1/2 c. coconut milk 3 c. water

- 15 oz. diced tomatoes 1 1/2 tablespoon tomato paste

- 8 oz. cremini mushrooms 2 zucchini, diced

- 2 green bell peppers, diced

- 2 chipotle peppers in adobo sauce, minced 1 ½ t. paprika

- 4 t. cumin

- 2 t. chili powder

- 1 1/2 t. cinnamon, ground 2 cloves garlic

- 5 stalks celery, diced

- 2 tablespoon extra-virgin olive oil

- Salt and pepper to taste

Directions:

1. Prepare the tofu by taking it out of the package and blotting with a paper towel until most of the moisture is gone.

2. Bring a skillet to medium heat; crumble the tofu and cook until browned.

3. In a big saucepan, heat the olive oil under medium heat, add celery, and cook for 4 minutes.

4. Add the celery, paprika, cumin, chili powder, cinnamon, and garlic and sauté for 2 minutes.

5. Next, add the mushrooms, zucchini, and bell peppers and cook for approximately 5 minutes.

6. In the big saucepan add cocoa powder, walnuts, tofu, coconut milk, water, tomatoes, tomato paste, and chipotle and simmer for 20-25 minutes or until thick.

7. Dust with some salt and pepper according to preference.

Nutrition: Calories: 294 Carbohydrates: 17.1 g Proteins: 10.6 g Fats: 23.7 g

CHAPTER 17:

NUTRIENT-PACKED PROTEIN SALAD RECIPES

38. Rice & Tofu Salad

Preparation Time: 15 Minutes

Cooking Time: 0 Minutes

Servings: 4

Ingredients:

Salad:

- 1 (12-ounce) package firm tofu, pressed, drained, and sliced
- 1½ cups cooked brown rice
- 3 large tomatoes, peeled and chopped
- ¼ cup fresh basil leaves

Dressing

- 3 scallions, chopped
- 2 tablespoons black sesame seeds, toasted
- 2 tablespoons low-sodium soy sauce
- ½ teaspoon sesame oil, toasted
- Drop of hot pepper sauce
- 1 tablespoon maple syrup
- ¼ teaspoon red chili powder

Directions:

1. In a large serving bowl, place all the Ingredients and toss to coat well.

2. Serve immediately.

Nutrition: Calories 393 Total Fat 8.6 g Cholesterol 0 mg Sodium 464 mg Total Carbs 66.9 g Fiber 5.7 g Sugar 7.9 g Protein 15.1 g

CHAPTER 18:

FINGER FOOD

39.   Pumpernickel with Avocado

Preparation Time: 10 minutes

Cooking Time: 0 minutes

Servings: 2

Ingredients:

- 6 small slices of pumpernickel
- 1 avocado
- 1 roll of vegan cheese spread
- 1 tablespoon chives
- Salt and pepper

Directions:

1. Halve the avocado, remove the seeds and carefully remove from the skin. Cut into slices and place on a plate.

2. Spread cheese on the bread, then top with avocado and then sprinkle with a little pepper and chopped chives.

Nutrition: Calories: 159 Fat: 9.4g Carbs: 10.5g Protein: 9.1g Fiber: 3.2g

CHAPTER 19:

FRUIT SALAD RECIPES

40. Fall Fruit with Creamy Dressing

Preparation Time: 25 Minutes

Cooking Time: 0 Minutes

Servings: 4

Ingredients:

Salad

- Pumpkin, raw, shredded, one half cup
- Pomegranate seeds, one half cup
- Grapes, one cup
- Apples, three, cored and cubed

Creamy Dressing

- Cinnamon, one teaspoon
- Lemon juice, one tablespoon
- Almond yogurt, one half cup

Directions:

1. Mix together all of the listed Ingredients for the dressing.

2. In a large-sized bowl, toss the dressing with the shredded raw pumpkin, pomegranate seeds, apples, and the dressing. Serve immediately.

Nutrition: Calories: 161 Protein: 3g Fat: 1g Carbs: 40g

CHAPTER 20:

GRAINS AND BEANS

41. Noodle and Rice Pilaf

Preparation Time: 5 minutes

Cooking Time: 33 to 44 minutes

Servings: 6 to 8

Ingredients:

- 1 cup whole-wheat noodles, broken into 1/8 inch pieces

- 2 cups long-grain brown rice

- 6½ cups low-sodium vegetable broth

- 1 teaspoon ground cumin

- ½ teaspoon dried oregano

Directions:

1. Combine the noodles and rice in a saucepan over medium heat and cook for 3 to 4 minutes, or until they begin to smell toasted.

2. Stir in the vegetable broth, cumin and oregano. Bring to a boil. Reduce the heat to medium-low. Cover and cook for 30 to 40 minutes, or until all water is absorbed.

Nutrition: calories: 287 fat: 2.5g carbs: 58.1g protein: 7.9g fiber: 5.0g

42. Easy Millet Loaf

Preparation Time: 5 minutes

Cooking Time: 1 hour 15 minutes

Servings: 4

Ingredients:

- 1¼ cups millet
- 4 cups unsweetened tomato juice
- 1 medium onion, chopped
- 1 to 2 cloves garlic
- ½ teaspoon dried sage
- ½ teaspoon dried basil
- ½ teaspoon poultry seasoning

Directions:

1. Preheat the oven to 350°F (180°C).
2. Place the millet in a large bowl.
3. Place the remaining ingredients in a blender and pulse until smooth. Add to the bowl with the millet and mix well.
4. Pour the mixture into a shallow casserole dish. Cover and bake in the oven for 1¼ hours, or until set.
5. Serve warm.

Nutrition: calories: 315 fat: 3.4g carbs: 61.6g protein: 10.2g fiber: 9.6g

CHAPTER 21:

DRINKS

43.   Turmeric Lassi

Preparation Time: 5 minutes   **Cooking Time:** 0 minute

Servings: 2

Ingredients:

- 1 teaspoon grated ginger
- 1/8 teaspoon ground black pepper
- 1 teaspoon turmeric powder
- 1/8 teaspoon cayenne
- 1 tablespoon coconut sugar
- 1/8 teaspoon salt
- 1 cup vegan yogurt
- 1 cup almond milk

Directions:

1. Place all the ingredients in the order in a food processor or blender and then pulse for 2 to 3 minutes at high speed until smooth.
2. Pour the lassi into two glasses and then serve.

Nutrition: Calories: 392 Fat: 10g Protein: 18g Sugar: 8g

44.   Brownie Batter Orange Chia Shake

Preparation Time: 5 minutes

Cooking Time: 0 minute

Servings: 2

Ingredients:

- 2 tablespoons cocoa powder
- 3 tablespoons chia seeds
- ¼ teaspoon salt
- 4 tablespoons chocolate chips
- 4 teaspoons coconut sugar
- ½ teaspoon orange zest
- ½ teaspoon vanilla extract, unsweetened
- 2 cup almond milk

Directions:

1. Place all the ingredients in the order in a food processor or blender and then pulse for 2 to 3 minutes at high speed until smooth.
2. Pour the smoothie into two glasses and then serve.

Nutrition: Calories: 290 Fat: 11g Protein: 20g Sugar: 9g

45. <u>Saffron Pistachio Beverage</u>

Preparation Time: 5 minutes

Cooking Time: 0 minute

Servings: 2

Ingredients:

- 8 strands of saffron
- 1 tablespoon cashews
- 1/4 teaspoon ground ginger
- 2 tablespoons pistachio
- 1/8 teaspoon cloves
- 1/4 teaspoon ground black pepper
- 1/4 teaspoon cardamom powder
- 3 tablespoons coconut sugar
- 1/4 teaspoon cinnamon
- 1/8 teaspoon fennel seeds
- 1/4 teaspoon poppy seeds

Directions:

1. Place all the ingredients in the order in a food processor or blender and then pulse for 2 to 3 minutes at high speed until smooth.
2. Pour the smoothie into two glasses and then serve.

Nutrition: Calories: 394 Fat: 5g Protein: 12g Sugar: 4g

CHAPTER 22:

DESSERTS

46.   Banana-Almond Cake

Preparation Time: 15 minutes

Cooking Time: 45 minutes

Servings: 8

Ingredients:

- 4 ripe bananas in chunks
- 3 Tbsš honey or maple syrup
- 1 tsp pure vanilla extract
- 1/2 cup almond milk
- 3/4 cup of self-raising flour
- 1 tsp cinnamon
- 1 tsp baking powder
- 1 pinch of salt
- 1/3 cup of almonds finely chopped
- Almond slices for decoration

Directions:

1. Preheat the oven to 400 F (air mode).
2. Oil a cake mold; set aside.

3. Add bananas into a bowl and mash with the fork.

4. Add honey, vanilla, almond, and stir well.

5. In a separate bowl, stir flour, cinnamon, baking powder, salt, the almonds broken, and mix with a spoon.

6. Combine the flour mixture with the banana mixture, and stir until all ingredients combined well.

7. Transfer the mixture to prepared cake mold and sprinkle with sliced almonds.

8. Bake for 40-45 minutes or until the toothpick inserted comes out clean.

9. Remove from the oven, and allow the cake to cool completely.

10. Cut cake into slices, place in tin foil, or an airtight container, and keep refrigerated up to one week.

Nutrition: Calories: 301 Total fat: 8g Saturated Fat: 1g Cholesterol: 99mg Sodium: 808mg Carbohydrates: 21g Fiber: 4g Protein: 26g

47. Banana-Coconut Ice Cream

Preparation Time: 15 minutes

Cooking Time: 0 minutes

Servings: 6

Ingredients:

- 1 cup coconut cream
- 1/2 cup Inverted sugar
- 2 large frozen bananas (chunks)
- 3 Tbsp honey extracted
- 1/4 tsp cinnamon powder

Directions:

1. In a bowl, whip the coconut cream with the inverted sugar.
2. In a separate bowl, beat the banana with honey and cinnamon.
3. Incorporate the coconut whipped cream and banana mixture; stir well.
4. Cover the bowl and let cool in the refrigerator over the night.
5. Stir the mixture 3 to 4 times to avoid crystallization.
6. Keep frozen 1 to 2 months.

Nutrition: Calories: 257 Total Fat: 4g Saturated Fat: 0g Cholesterol: 33mg Sodium: 819mg Carbohydrates: 37g Fiber: 7g Protein: 20g

48. Coconut Butter Clouds Cookies

Preparation Time: 15 minutes

Cooking Time: 10 minutes

Servings: 8

Ingredients:

- 1/2 cup coconut butter softened
- 1/2 cup peanut butter softened
- 1/2 cup of granulated sugar
- 1/2 cup of brown sugar
- 2 Tbsp chia seeds soaked in 4 tablespoons water
- 1/2 tsp pure vanilla extract
- 1/2 tsp baking soda
- 1/4 tsp salt
- 1 cup of all-purpose flour

Directions:

1. Preheat oven to 360 F.
2. Add coconut butter, peanut butter, and both sugars in a mixing bowl.
3. Beat with a mixer until soft and sugar combined well.
4. Add soaked chia seeds and vanilla extract; beat.
5. Add baking soda, salt, and flour; beat until all ingredients are combined well.
6. With your hands, shape dough into cookies.
7. Arrange your cookies onto a baking sheet, and bake for about 10 minutes.

8. Remove cookies from the oven and allow to cool completely.

9. Sprinkle with icing sugar and enjoy your cookies.

10. Place cookies in an airtight container and keep refrigerated up to 10 days.

Nutrition: Calories: 731 Total Fat: 26g Saturated Fat: 17g Cholesterol: 169mg Sodium: 1167mg Carbohydrates: 56g Fiber: 5g Protein: 45g

49.   Chocomint Hazelnut Bars

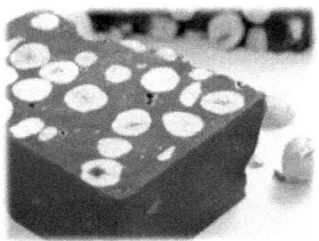

Preparation Time: 5 minutes

Cooking Time: 15 minutes

Servings: 8

Ingredients:

- 1/2 cup coconut oil, melted
- 4 Tbsp cocoa powder
- 1/4 cup almond butter
- 3/4 cup brown sugar - (packed)
- 1 tsp vanilla extract
- 1 tsp pure peppermint extract
- pinch of salt
- 1 cup shredded coconut
- 1 cup hazelnuts sliced

Directions:

1. Chop the hazelnuts in a food processor; set aside.

2. Fill the bottom of a double boiler with water and place it on low heat.

3. Put the coconut oil, cacao powder, almond butter, brown sugar, vanilla, peppermint extract, and salt in the top of a

double boiler over hot (not boiling) water and constantly stir for 10 minutes.

4. Add hazelnuts and shredded coconut to the melted mixture and stir together.

5. Pour the mixture in a dish lined with parchment and freeze for several hours.

6. Remove from the freezer and cut into bars.

7. Store in airtight container or freezer bag in a freezer.

8. Let the bars at room temperature for 10 to 15 minutes before eating.

Nutrition: Calories: 186 Total Fat: 4g Saturated Fat: 0g Cholesterol: 33mg Sodium: 783mg Carbohydrates: 23g Fiber: 6g Protein: 19g

50.   Coco-Cinnamon Balls

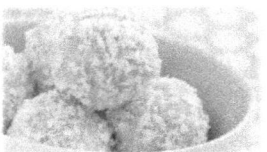

Preparation Time: 10 minutes

Cooking Time: 5 minutes

Servings: 12

Ingredients:

- 1 cup coconut butter softened
- 1 cup coconut milk canned
- 1 tsp pure vanilla extract
- 3/4 tsp cinnamon
- 1/2 tsp nutmeg
- 2 Tbsp coconut palm sugar (or granulated sugar)
- 1 cup coconut shreds

Directions:

1. Combine all ingredients (except the coconut shreds) in a heated bath - bain-marie.
2. Cook and stir until all ingredients are soft and well combined.
3. Remove bowl from heat, place into a bowl, and refrigerate until the mixture firmed up.
4. Form cold coconut mixture into balls, and roll each ball in the shredded coconut.

5. Store into a sealed container, and keep refrigerated up to one week.

Nutrition: Calories: 213 Fat: 6g Fiber: 13g Carbs: 16g Protein: 22g

CHAPTER 23:

2 WEEKS MEAL PLAN

Day	Breakfast	Lunch	Dinner	Dessert/snacks
1	Gingerbread Waffles	Chickpea Sunflower Sandwich	Black Bean Burgers	Express Coconut Flax Pudding
2	Oatmeal & Peanut Butter Breakfast Bar	Pesto Quinoa with White Beans	Dijon Maple Burgers	Pumpkin Pie Cups
3	Easy Hummus Toast	White Bean and Artichoke Sandwich	Bok Choy Salad	Banana-Coconut Ice Cream
4	Blueberry French Toast Breakfast Muffins	Rainbow Taco Boats	Garlic Zucchini and Cauliflower	Nice Spiced Cherry Cider
5	Avocado Toast with White Beans	Green Bean Casserole	Herbed Beets	Full-flavored Vanilla Ice Cream
6	Sweet Pomegranate Porridge	Roasted Vegetables	Spinach and Pear Salad	Strawberry Coconut Ice Cream
7	Vegan Breakfast Biscuits	Loaded Kale Salad	Steamed Cauliflower	Roasted Almond Protein Salad
8	Orange French Toast	Mediterranean Pizza	Olives and Mango Mix	Dark Chocolate Bars
9	Coffee Smoothie	Pumpkin Risotto	Marinara Broccoli	Mimosa Salad
10	Berries and Banana	Black Bean and Quinoa	Red Onion, Avocado	Mixed Berries and Cream

	Smoothie Bowl	Salad	and Radishes Mix	
11	Carrot Cake Oats	Spicy Peanut Soba Noodles	Sage Walnuts and Radishes	Pear Lemonade
12	Dairy-Free Coconut Yogurt	Tahini Broccoli	Curried Apple	Brownie Energy Bites
13	Mint Chocolate Green Protein	Garden Pasta Salad	Cajun and Balsamic Okra	Beetroot Hummus
14	Cinnamon Rolls with Cashew Frosting	Jamaican Jerk Tofu Wrap	Plant Based Keto Lo Mein	Skewers of Mozzarella And Tomato

CONCLUSION

In a nutshell, this cookbook offers you a world full of options to diversify your plant-based menu. People on this diet are usually seen struggling to choose between healthy food and flavor but, soon, they run out of the options. The selection of 250 recipes in this book is enough to adorn your dinner table with flavorsome, plant-based meals every day. Give each recipe a good read and try them out in the kitchen. You will experience tempting aromas and binding flavors every day.

The book is conceptualized with the idea of offering you a comprehensive view of a plant-based diet and how it can benefit the body. You may find the shift sudden, especially if you are a die-hard fan of non-vegetarian items. But you need not give up anything that you love. Eat everything in moderation.

The next step is to start experimenting with the different recipes in this book and see which ones are your favorites. Everyone has their favorite food, and you will surely find several of yours in this book. Start with breakfast and work your way through. You will be pleasantly surprised at how tasty a vegan meal really can be.

You will love reading this book, as it helps you to understand how revolutionary a plant-based diet can be. It will help you to make informed decisions as you move toward greater change for the greater good. What are you waiting for? Have you begun your journey on the path of the plant-based diet yet? If you haven't, do it now!

Now you have everything you need to get started making budget-friendly, healthy plant-based recipes. Just follow your basic shopping list and follow your meal plan to get started! It's easy to switch over to a plant-based diet if you have your meals planned out and temptation locked away. Don't forget to clean out your kitchen before starting, and you're sure to meet all your diet and health goals.

You need to plan if you are thinking about dieting. First, you can start slowly by just eating one meal a day, which is vegetarian and gradually increasing your number of vegetarian meals. Whenever you are struggling, ask your friend or family member to support you and keep you motivated. One important thing is also to be regularly accountable for not following the diet.

If dieting seems very important to you and you need to do it right, then it is recommended that you visit a professional such as a nutritionist or dietitian to discuss your dieting plan and optimizing it for the better.

No matter how much you want to lose weight, it is not advised that you decrease your calorie intake to an unhealthy level. Losing weight does not mean that you stop eating. It is done by carefully planning meals.

A plant-based diet is very easy once you get into it. At first, you will start to face a lot of difficulties, but if you start slowly, then you can face all the barriers and achieve your goal.

Swap out one unhealthy food item each week that you know is not helping you and put in its place one of the plant-based ingredients that you like. Then have some fun creating the many different recipes in this book. Find out what recipes you like the most so you can make them often and most of all; have some fun exploring all your recipe options.

Wish you good luck with the plant-based diet!

CPSIA information can be obtained
at www.ICGtesting.com
Printed in the USA
LVHW021117120221
679116LV00003B/704